Table of Contents

0-6 Pack Abs Disclaimer

By Tyler J. Bramlett

Manufactured in the United States of America
Published by: Warrior Media, Inc., Santa Cruz, California

DISCLAIMER STATEMENT: Exercise, Nutrition and Lifestyle books and videos sold and distributed by Warrior Media, Inc., or it's partners or partnered websites reflects the authors personal experience and is provided for educational purposes and general reference. This is not to be used as a substitute for medical advice or counseling.

The reader assumes all risks from the use, non-use or misuse of the book. Neither the author or publisher assumes any responsibility for the use or misuse of the information contained in this book. Please consult a Physician before beginning any nutrition and exercise program.

Introduction

First of all... CONGRATULATIONS!

You now have in your hands the greatest ab training system ever developed! And...

While this may seem like a bold claim, I'm 100% positive that after going through the Phase 1 system that was developed by Dr. James Vegher and the Phase 2 system that was developed by me, you'll agree that this is the best ab training system ever created.

We laid this manual out into 2 sections, Phase 1 and Phase 2 each with their own intro and basic outline of how to use the system.

For best results I highly recommend that you use the follow-along videos. This way you can stay motivated during your workouts and make sure your form is perfect. Finally...

It's very likely that you are going to want to skip the Phase 1 system. After all, the exercises are going to seem strangely easy. But PLEASE! Stick with it because Dr. James Vegher's Phase 1 exercises are **THE KEY** to making this system work!

Let's dive right in and have you go over the 4 steps to using the Phase 1 system...

PHASE I

How to Use Phase 1 Workouts

All you have to do to get amazing results with the Phase 1 part of the program is follow the 4 steps below...

STEP#1 - Look through the Phase 1 workouts and exercises below to become familiar with this part of the system.

STEP#2 - Regardless of how strong your think your core is, start off by following along to the Phase 1 Level 1 workout video. If you prefer not to follow along to the video, you can refer to the exercises from the Level 1 workout in the manual and practice each one for roughly 60-90 seconds. For best results, follow along to the video with Dr. James Vegher.

STEP#3 - After you finish each exercise in the workout, score how well you did on the exercise based on how easy it was to do. 10 meaning that it was extremely easy and 1 meaning that it was hard!

STEP#4 - Repeat the Phase 1 Level 1 workout a minimum of 3 days a week (It can be done daily if you wish) until you feel you have earned a score of a 9 or above on ever exercises.

STEP#5 - After you complete the Phase 1 Level 1 workout with perfect form during the whole workout, move to the Phase 1 Level 2 Workout and repeat Steps 2-5

NOTE: Once you complete the Phase 1 Level 4 workout, go to Phase 2 and make sure to practice Phase 1 Level 4 a minimum of once a week to maintain your connection with your core.

PHASE I
WORKOUTS

PHASE 1 WORKOUT 1

You can do each exercise for 30-45 seconds. For best results follow along to the Phase 1 Level 1 video.

LEVEL 1

- Birthday Candles
- Elevator
- Arm Flexion
- Head Raise
- Rolling

YOUR SCORE SHEET

Birthday Candles	
Elevator	
Arm Flexion	
Head Raise	
Rolling	

PHASE 1 WORKOUT 2

You can do each exercise for 30-45 seconds. For best results follow along to the Phase 1 Level 2 video.

LEVEL 2

- Birthday Candles
- Tin Soldier
- Leg Raise w/ Arm Flexion
- Head Raise
- Arm and Leg Raise
- Arm and Leg Raise w/ Flexion
- Pelvic Lift
- Foot Grab

YOUR SCORE SHEET

Birthday Candles	
Tin Soldier	
Leg Raise with Arm Flexion	
Head Raise	
Arm and Leg Raise	
Arm and Leg Raise with Flexion	
Pelvic Lift	
Foot Grab	

PHASE 1 WORKOUT 3

You can do each exercise for 30-45 seconds. For best results follow along to the Phase 1 Level 3 video.

LEVEL 3

- Leg Raise
- 3 Month Position
- Arm and Leg Raise
- Tin Soldier
- Head Raise
- Foot Grab
- Oyster

YOUR SCORE SHEET

Leg Raise	
3 Month Position	
Arm and Leg Raise	
Tin Soldier	
Head Raise	
Foot Grab	
Oyster	

PHASE 1 WORKOUT 4

You can do each exercise for 30-45 seconds. For best results follow along to the Phase 1 Level 4 video.

LEVEL 4

- Birthday Candles
- 3 Month Position
- Rolling
- Arm and Leg Raise with Flexion
- Tin Soldier
- Pelvic Lift
- Foot Grab
- Happy Baby
- Oyster

YOUR SCORE SHEET

Birthday Candles	
3 Month Position	
Rolling	
Arm and Leg Raise with Flexion	
Tin Soldier	
Pelvic Lift	
Foot Grab	
Happy Baby	
Oyster	

PHASE I
EXERCISES

BIRTHDAY CANDLES

Step 1

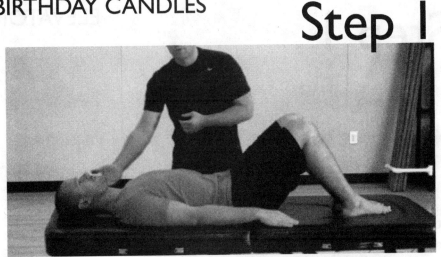

Start by lying on your back with your knees bent, arms by your side and your head lying flat.

Step 2

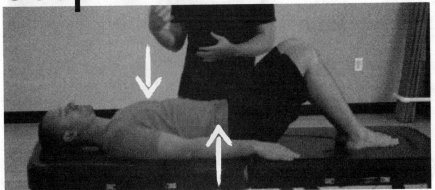

Breath in and out, focusing on allowing your ribs to drop down while filling your belly with air. Exhale slowly, letting your ribs drop slowly, like you are trying to blow out birthday candles.

Step 1

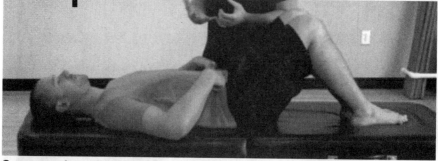

Start in the same position as in *Birthday Candles*. Lie on your back, with your knees bent, but now bring your hands to your pelvis 1/2 way between your belly button and hip bone.

Step 2

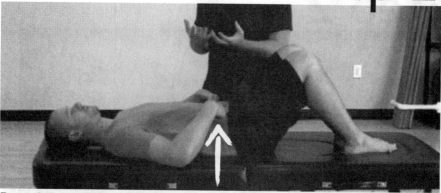

Breathe in and out, trying the whole time to push out against your hands as if you were trying push them to the top floor of a 10 story building. Remember to allow your ribs to drop down as you exhale.

Step 1

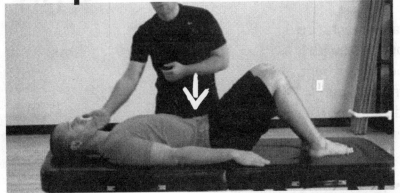

Begin lying down with your arms by your sides and your knees bent. Engage your *"Elevator"* to floor 5 before beginning the movement.

Step 2

Maintaining your 5th floor elevator, bring your knee and your arm up at the same time. Your palm should be facing the ground and your hips should be inline. Repeat with the other side.

ARM FLEXION

Start, by lying on your back with your knees bent, arms by your side and your head lying flat.

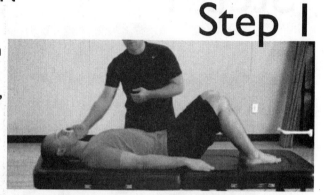

Step 1

Step 2

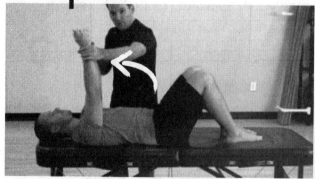

Raise your *"Elevator"* to around the 5th floor and lift your arms in front of your face with your palms facing each other.

Step 3

Bring your arms further above your head. Still dropping your ribs down and keeping your *"Elevator"* to around the 5th floor.

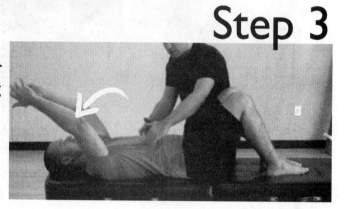

LEG FLEXION

Step 1

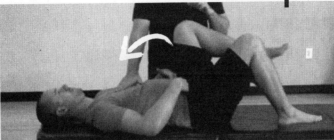

This position starts the same as the prior movements. Hold your 5th floor *"Elevator"*. While in this position, bring your left knee up and to the outside. This ensures your hips remain in the proper alignment with your core.

Step 2

Return to the start and repeat with the other knee. Make sure your hips are staying in line with your core the entire time.

Step 3

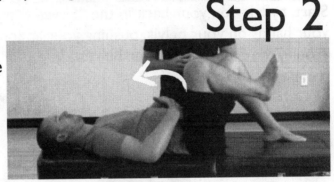

When you have become proficient in the first two, you may pick up both knees at the same time.

Step 1

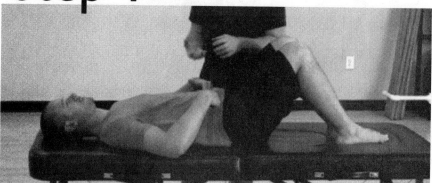

Start, by lying on your back in the *"Elevator"* position, with your hands on your pelvis, pushing your abdomen out to around the 5th floor of your building.

Step 2

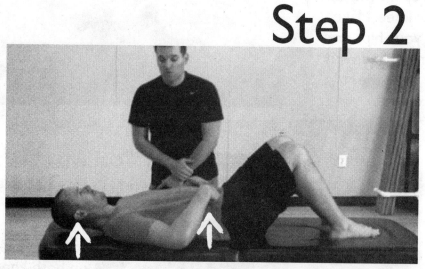

From that initial position, lift your head without moving any other part of you body and maintaing that 5th floor pressure.

Step 1

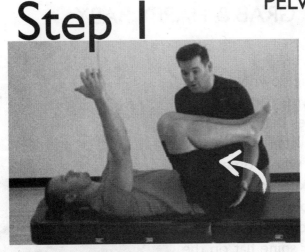

Begin lying down with your arms by your sides and your knees bent. Engage your *"Elevator"* to the 5th floor before beginning the movement. Bring your arms and your knees up to the ceiling.

Step 2

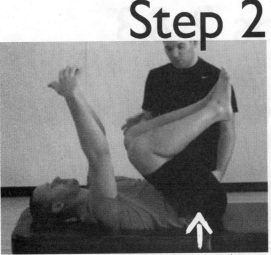

From that position, lift your pelvis off the ground and think about pushing your knees to the sky. You will feel this more than actually see it. Hold for a few seconds and repeat making sure you keep your *"Elevator"* at the 5th floor.

FOOT GRAB & HAPPY BABY

Step 1

Begin lying down with your arms by your sides and your knees bent. Activate your *"Elevator"* to the 5th floor the whole time you do this exercise. Bring your feet to your hands and your hands to your feet with your spine flat on the ground.

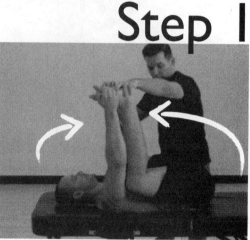

Steps 2 &3

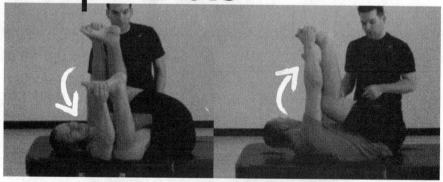

From the foot grab position, begin the *Happy Baby* by rolling side to side. Making sure there is no flexion of the spine.

Variation 1

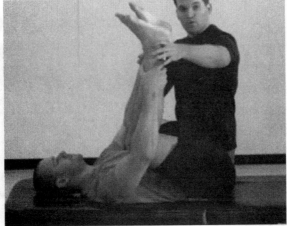

If you do not quite have flexible enough hips to get into the *Foot Grab*, then you may grab lower down your calf.

Variation 2

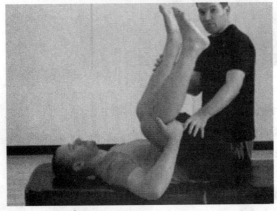

If grabbing your calf still poses a challenge, then you may grab right behind your hamstrings. Remember the goal is not strength, it is coordination.

OYSTER

Start by lying on your back with your knees bent, arms by your side and your head lying flat. Engage your *"Elevator"* to the 5th floor and bring your knees to your chest.

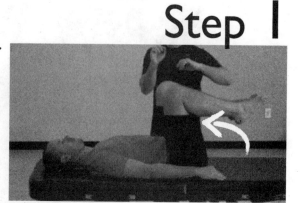

Step 1

Step 2

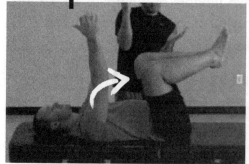

From there, bring your arms up to meet your knees.

Step 3

Then reach your arms through your knees. Maintain your 5th floor elevator and raise your pelvis up to the ceiling.

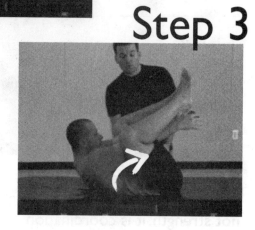

Step 1

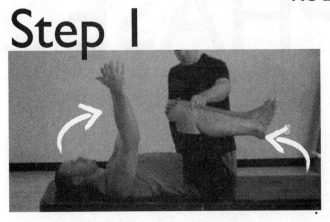

Bring your knees and arms up the the sky. Knees should be apart and your 5th floor *"Elevator"* should be engaged. Make sure you keep your spine pressed to the floor.

Step 2

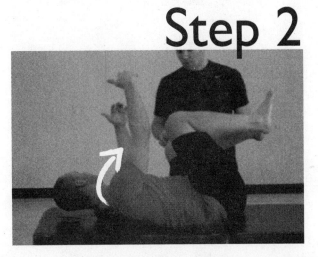

Roll slowly from side to side making sure there is no flexion of the spine and that the hips and shoulders are moving simultaneously.

PHASE 2

How to Use Phase 2 Workouts

All you have to do to get amazing results with the Phase 2 part of the program is follow the 6 steps below...

STEP#1 - Look through the Phase 2 workouts and exercises below to become familiar with this part of the system.

STEP#2 - Regardless of how strong your think your core is, start off by following along to the Phase 2 Level 1 Workout 1 video after your regular workout. If you prefer not to follow along to the video, you can refer to the exercises from Level 1 Workout 1 in the manual and follow along using an interval timer for the prescribed time. For best results, follow along to the video with me so I can help keep you motivated and your form perfect.

STEP#3 - After you complete the Phase 2 Level 1 Workout 1 with perfect form on every rep or hold, move to Phase 2 Level 1 Workout 2 and follow the Phase 2 system a minimum of 3 days and a maximum of 5 days a week.

NOTE: If you fail to do the workout with perfect form, simply give yourself a days rest and try it again the next day.

STEP#4 - After you complete the Phase 2 Level 1 Workout 2 with perfect form on every rep or hold, move to Phase 2 Level 1 Workout 3.

STEP#5 - After you complete the Phase 2 Level 1 Workout 3 with perfect form on every rep or hold, move to Phase 2 Level 1 Workout 4.

STEP#6 - After you complete the Phase 2 Level 1 Workout 4 with perfect form on every rep or hold, move to Phase 2 Level 2 Workout 1.

That's it! Let's get started with these Phase 2 Level 1 workouts...

PHASE 2
LEVEL 1
WORKOUTS
AND
EXERCISES

LEVEL 1 WORKOUT 1

WORKOUT

- Kneeling Plank
- :40 seconds of WORK/ :20 seconds of REST
- Bent Knee Alternating Lying Leg Raises **(Hands Under Butt)**
- :40 seconds of WORK/ :20 seconds REST

TRACK YOUR WORKOUT

Rounds	Kneeling Plank	Bent Knee Alternating Lying Leg Raises
1		

HOW TO SCORE YOUR WORKOUT: Score this workout by ranking each exercise and set on a scale of 1-10 (10 being you performed every rep with perfect form for the entire 40 second interval). Once you have a 9 or 10 on every round, move on to the **next workout.**

LEVEL 1 WORKOUT 2

WORKOUT

- Kneeling Plank
- :40 seconds of WORK/ :20 seconds of REST
- Bent Knee Alternating Lying Leg Raises **(Hands Under Butt)**
- :40 seconds of WORK/ :20 seconds REST

TRACK YOUR WORKOUT

Rounds	Kneeling Plank	Bent Knee Alternating Lying Leg Raises
1		
2		

HOW TO SCORE YOUR WORKOUT: Score this workout by ranking each exercise and set on a scale of 1-10 (10 being you performed every rep with perfect form for the entire 40 second interval). Once you have a 9 or 10 on every round, move on to the next workout.

LEVEL I WORKOUT 3

WORKOUT

Kneeling Plank
- :40 seconds of WORK/ :20 seconds of REST
Bent Knee Alternating Lying Leg Raises **(Hands Under Butt)**
- :40 seconds of WORK/ :20 seconds REST

TRACK YOUR WORKOUT

Rounds	Kneeling Plank	Bent Knee Alternating Lying Leg Raises
1		
2		
3		

HOW TO SCORE YOUR WORKOUT: Score this workout by ranking each exercise and set on a scale of 1-10 (10 being you performed every rep with perfect form for the entire 40 second interval). Once you have a 9 or 10 on every round, move on to the next workout.

LEVEL I WORKOUT 4

WORKOUT

Kneeling Plank
- :40 seconds of WORK/ :20 seconds of REST

Bent Knee Alternating Lying Leg Raises **(Hands Under Butt)**
- :40 seconds of WORK/ :20 seconds REST

TRACK YOUR WORKOUT

Rounds	Kneeling Plank	Bent Knee Alternating Lying Leg Raises
1		
2		
3		
4		

HOW TO SCORE YOUR WORKOUT: Score this workout by ranking each exercise and set on a scale of 1-10 (10 being you performed every rep with perfect form for the entire 40 second interval). Once you have a 9 or 10 on every round, move on to the next workout.

Step 1

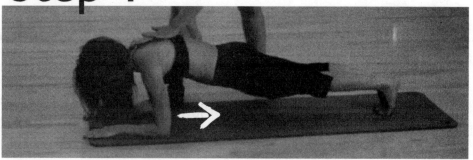

Start in a kneeling plank and bring both your knees off the ground so toes and elbows are supporting your weight. Remember to squeeze your core, butt and lats while driving your elbows down.

ALTERNATING BENT KNEE LYING LEG RAISES

Step 1

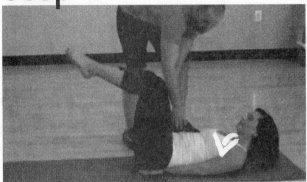

Start lying on your back and bring your hands underneath your butt. Squeeze your core and bring your knees to your chest at around a 90° angle. From here alternate touching each foot to the ground.

Step 2 & 3

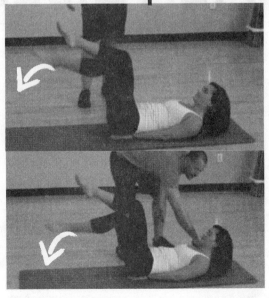

PHASE 2
LEVEL 2
WORKOUTS
AND
EXERCISES

LEVEL 2 WORKOUT 1

WORKOUT

½ Kneeling Plank
- 20 sec LEFT + 20 sec RIGHT **WORK**/ 20 sec REST
Bent Knee Lying Leg Raises **(Hands Under Butt)**
- 40 sec of WORK/ 20 sec REST

TRACK YOUR WORKOUT

Rounds	½ Kneeling Plank LEFT	½ Kneeling Plank RIGHT	Bent Knee Lying Leg Raises
1			

HOW TO SCORE YOUR WORKOUT: Score this workout by ranking each exercise and set on a scale of 1-10 (10 being you performed every rep with perfect form for the entire 40 second interval). Once you have a 9 or 10 on every round, move on to the next workout.

LEVEL 2 WORKOUT 2

WORKOUT

½ Kneeling Plank
- 20 sec LEFT + 20 sec RIGHT **WORK**/ 20 sec REST
Bent Knee Lying Leg Raises **(Hands Under Butt)**
- 40 sec of WORK/ 20 sec REST

TRACK YOUR WORKOUT

Rounds	½ Kneeling Plank LEFT	½ Kneeling Plank RIGHT	Bent Knee Lying Leg Raises
1			
2			

HOW TO SCORE YOUR WORKOUT: Score this workout by ranking each exercise and set on a scale of 1-10 (10 being you performed every rep with perfect form for the entire 40 second interval). Once you have a 9 or 10 on every round, move on to the next workout.

LEVEL 2 WORKOUT 3

WORKOUT

½ Kneeling Plank
- 20 sec LEFT + 20 sec RIGHT **WORK**/ 20 sec REST
Bent Knee Lying Leg Raises **(Hands Under Butt)**
- 40 sec of WORK/ 20 sec REST

TRACK YOUR WORKOUT

Rounds	½ Kneeling Plank LEFT	½ Kneeling Plank RIGHT	Bent Knee Lying Leg Raises
1			
2			
3			

HOW TO SCORE YOUR WORKOUT: Score this workout by ranking each exercise and set on a scale of 1-10 (10 being you performed every rep with perfect form for the entire 40 second interval). Once you have a 9 or 10 on every round, move on to the next workout.

LEVEL 2 WORKOUT 4

WORKOUT

½ Kneeling Plank
- 20 sec LEFT + 20 sec RIGHT **WORK**/ 20 sec REST
Bent Knee Lying Leg Raises **(Hands Under Butt)**
- 40 sec of WORK/ 20 sec REST

TRACK YOUR WORKOUT

Rounds	½ Kneeling Plank LEFT	½ Kneeling Plank RIGHT	Bent Knee Lying Leg Raises
1			
2			
3			
4			

HOW TO SCORE YOUR WORKOUT: Score this workout by ranking each exercise and set on a scale of 1-10 (10 being you performed every rep with perfect form for the entire 40 second interval). Once you have a 9 or 10 on every round, move on to the next workout.

LEVEL 2 WORKOUT 4

WORKOUT

½ Kneeling Plank
- 20 sec LEFT + 20 sec RIGHT **WORK**/ 20 sec REST
Bent Knee Lying Leg Raises **(Hands Under Butt)**
- 40 sec of WORK/ 20 sec REST

TRACK YOUR WORKOUT

Rounds	½ Kneeling Plank LEFT	½ Kneeling Plank RIGHT	Bent Knee Lying Leg Raises
1			
2			
3			
4			

HOW TO SCORE YOUR WORKOUT: Score this workout by ranking each exercise and set on a scale of 1-10 (10 being you performed every rep with perfect form for the entire 40 second interval). Once you have a 9 or 10 on every round, move on to the next workout.

1/2 KNEELING KNEELING PLANK

Step 1

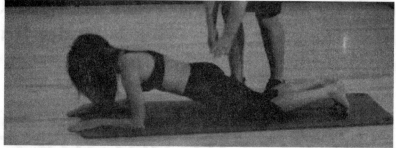

Start in a kneeling plank. Remember to squeeze your core, butt and lats. Also, pull you elbows down towards your knees.

Step 2

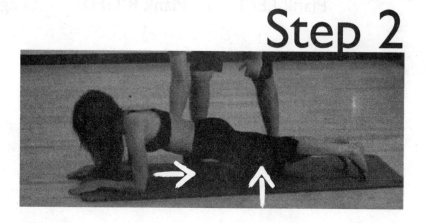

Pick one leg off the ground so only one leg is supporting your body.

BENT KNEE LYING LEG RAISE

Step 1

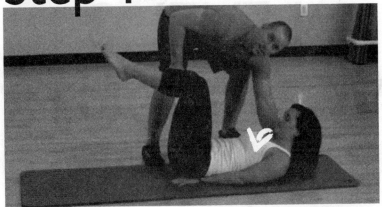

Start in the same lying position at the alternating bent knee leg raises. Squeeze your core and tuck your chin to your chest.

Step 2

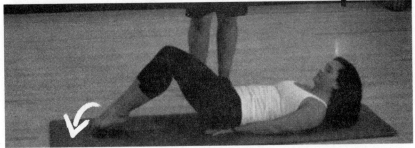

Lower both legs at the same time and tap your feet on the ground.

PHASE 2
LEVEL 3
WORKOUTS
AND
EXERCISES

LEVEL 3 WORKOUT 1

WORKOUT

Plank
- 40 sec WORK/ 20 sec REST

Alternating Lying Leg Raises **(Hands Under Butt)**
- 40 sec of WORK/ 20 sec REST

TRACK YOUR WORKOUT

Rounds	Plank	Alternating Lying Leg Raises
1		

HOW TO SCORE YOUR WORKOUT: Score this workout by ranking each exercise and set on a scale of 1-10 (10 being you performed every rep with perfect form for the entire 40 second interval). Once you have a 9 or 10 on every round, move on to the next workout.

LEVEL 3 WORKOUT 2

WORKOUT

Plank
- 40 sec WORK/ 20 sec REST

Alternating Lying Leg Raises **(Hands Under Butt)**
- 40 sec of WORK/ 20 sec REST

TRACK YOUR WORKOUT

Rounds	Plank	Alternating Lying Leg Raises
1		
2		

HOW TO SCORE YOUR WORKOUT: Score this workout by ranking each exercise and set on a scale of 1-10 (10 being you performed every rep with perfect form for the entire 40 second interval). Once you have a 9 or 10 on every round, move on to the next workout.

LEVEL 3 WORKOUT 3

WORKOUT

Plank
- 40 sec WORK/ 20 sec REST

Alternating Lying Leg Raises **(Hands Under Butt)**
- 40 sec of WORK/ 20 sec REST

TRACK YOUR WORKOUT

Rounds	Plank	Alternating Lying Leg Raises
1		
2		
3		

HOW TO SCORE YOUR WORKOUT: Score this workout by ranking each exercise and set on a scale of 1-10 (10 being you performed every rep with perfect form for the entire 40 second interval). Once you have a 9 or 10 on every round, move on to the next workout.

LEVEL 3 WORKOUT 4

WORKOUT

Plank
- 40 sec WORK/ 20 sec REST

Alternating Lying Leg Raises **(Hands Under Butt)**
- 40 sec of WORK/ 20 seconds REST

TRACK YOUR WORKOUT

Rounds	Plank	Alternating Lying Leg Raises
1		
2		
3		
4		

HOW TO SCORE YOUR WORKOUT: Score this workout by ranking each exercise and set on a scale of 1-10 (10 being you performed every rep with perfect form for the entire 40 second interval). Once you have a 9 or 10 on every round, move on to the next workout.

Step 1

Start in a kneeling plank and bring both your knees off the ground so toes and elbows are supporting your weight. Remember to squeeze your core, butt and lats while driving your elbows down.

ALTERNATING LYING LEG RAISE
HANDS UNDER BUTT

Step 1

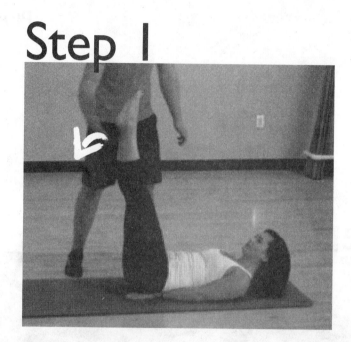

Start lying on your back with your hands under your butt. Squeeze your core and bring your legs up so they are completely straight in the air. From there alternate bringing each leg down to the ground.

Step 2& 3

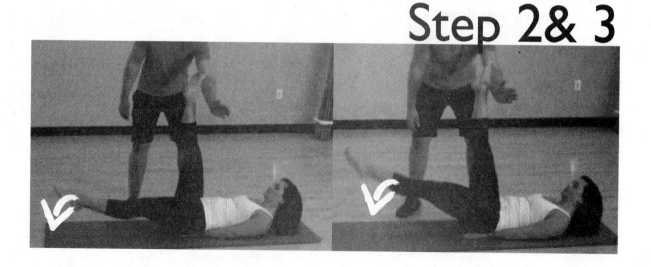

PHASE 2
LEVEL 4
WORKOUTS
AND
EXERCISES

LEVEL 4 WORKOUT 1

WORKOUT

One Leg Plank
- 40 sec LEFT + 20 sec RIGHT **WORK**/ 20 sec REST

Lying Leg Raises **(Hands Under Butt)**
- 40 sec of WORK/ 20 sec REST

TRACK YOUR WORKOUT

Rounds	One Leg Plank LEFT	One Leg Plank RIGHT	Lying Leg Raises
1			

HOW TO SCORE YOUR WORKOUT: Score this workout by ranking each exercise and set on a scale of 1-10 (10 being you performed every rep with perfect form for the entire 40 second interval). Once you have a 9 or 10 on every round, move on to the next workout.

LEVEL 4 WORKOUT 2

WORKOUT

One Leg Plank
- 40 sec LEFT + 20 sec RIGHT **WORK**/ 20 sec REST
Lying Leg Raises **(Hands Under Butt)**
- 40 sec of WORK/ 20 sec REST

TRACK YOUR WORKOUT

Rounds	One Leg Plank LEFT	One Leg Plank RIGHT	Lying Leg Raises
1			
2			

HOW TO SCORE YOUR WORKOUT: Score this workout by ranking each exercise and set on a scale of 1-10 (10 being you performed every rep with perfect form for the entire 40 second interval). Once you have a 9 or 10 on every round, move on to the next workout.

LEVEL 4 WORKOUT 3

WORKOUT

One Leg Plank
- 40 sec LEFT + 20 sec RIGHT **WORK**/ 20 sec REST

Lying Leg Raises **(Hands Under Butt)**
- 40 sec of WORK/ 20 sec REST

TRACK YOUR WORKOUT

Rounds	One Leg Plank LEFT	One Leg Plank RIGHT	Lying Leg Raises
1			
2			
3			

HOW TO SCORE YOUR WORKOUT: Score this workout by ranking each exercise and set on a scale of 1-10 (10 being you performed every rep with perfect form for the entire 40 second interval). Once you have a 9 or 10 on every round, move on to the next workout.

LEVEL 4 WORKOUT 4

WORKOUT

One Leg Plank
- 40 sec LEFT + 20 sec RIGHT **WORK**/ 20 sec REST
Lying Leg Raises **(Hands Under Butt)**
- 40 sec of WORK/ 20 sec REST

TRACK YOUR WORKOUT

Rounds	One Leg Plank LEFT	One Leg Plank RIGHT	Lying Leg Raises
1			
2			
3			
4			

HOW TO SCORE YOUR WORKOUT: Score this workout by ranking each exercise and set on a scale of 1-10 (10 being you performed every rep with perfect form for the entire 40 second interval). Once you have a 9 or 10 on every round, move on to the next workout.

ONE LEG PLANK

Step 1

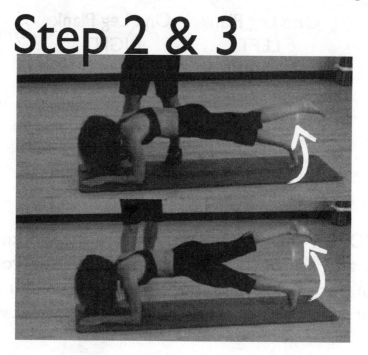

Start in a perfect plank, squeezing your core, butt and lats while driving your elbows down. While maintaining your plank, pick one leg off the ground. Hold and switch legs.

Step 2 & 3

LYING LEG RAISE
HANDS UNDER BUTT

Step 1

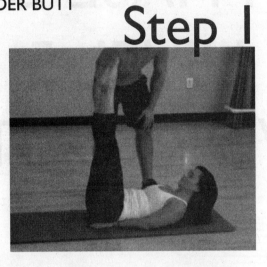

Start lying on your back with your hands tucked under your butt. Squeeze your core and bring your legs straight into the air.

Step 2

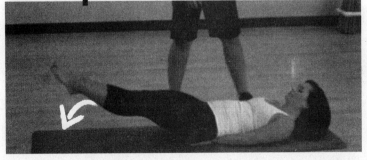

Bring both legs down at the same time while maintaining a tight core.

PHASE 2
LEVEL 5
WORKOUTS
AND
EXERCISES

LEVEL 5 WORKOUT I

WORKOUT

Swiss Ball Plank
- 40 sec WORK/ 20 sec REST
Alternating Lying Leg Raises **(Hands by Hips)**
- 40 sec of WORK/ 20 sec REST

TRACK YOUR WORKOUT

Rounds	Swiss Ball Plank	Alternating Lying Leg Raises
I		

HOW TO SCORE YOUR WORKOUT: Score this workout by ranking each exercise and set on a scale of 1-10 (10 being you performed every rep with perfect form for the entire 40 second interval). Once you have a 9 or 10 on every round, move on to the next workout.

LEVEL 5 WORKOUT 2

WORKOUT

Swiss Ball Plank
- 40 sec WORK/ 20 sec REST

Alternating Lying Leg Raises **(Hands by Hips)**
- 40 sec of WORK/ 20 sec REST

TRACK YOUR WORKOUT

Rounds	Swiss Ball Plank	Alternating Lying Leg Raises
1		
2		

HOW TO SCORE YOUR WORKOUT: Score this workout by ranking each exercise and set on a scale of 1-10 (10 being you performed every rep with perfect form for the entire 40 second interval). Once you have a 9 or 10 on every round, move on to the next workout.

LEVEL 5 WORKOUT 3

WORKOUT

Swiss Ball Plank
- 40 sec WORK/ 20 sec REST

Alternating Lying Leg Raises **(Hands by Hips)**
- 40 sec of WORK/ 20 sec REST

TRACK YOUR WORKOUT

Rounds	Swiss Ball Plank	Alternating Lying Leg Raises
1		
2		
3		

HOW TO SCORE YOUR WORKOUT: Score this workout by ranking each exercise and set on a scale of 1-10 (10 being you performed every rep with perfect form for the entire 40 second interval). Once you have a 9 or 10 on every round, move on to the next workout.

LEVEL 5 WORKOUT 4

WORKOUT

Swiss Ball Plank
- 40 sec WORK/ 20 sec REST

Alternating Lying Leg Raises **(Hands by Hips)**
- 40 sec of WORK/ 20 sec REST

TRACK YOUR WORKOUT

Rounds	Swiss Ball Plank	Alternating Lying Leg Raises
1		
2		
3		
4		

HOW TO SCORE YOUR WORKOUT: Score this workout by ranking each exercise and set on a scale of 1-10 (10 being you performed every rep with perfect form for the entire 40 second interval). Once you have a 9 or 10 on every round, move on to the next workout.

Step 1

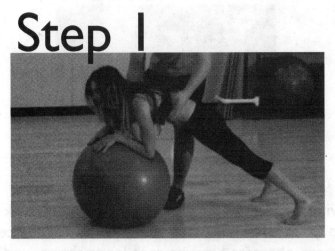

Start with your elbows on your swiss ball with your feel out wide for balance. Keep the same tightness as you would with a regular plank.

Step 2

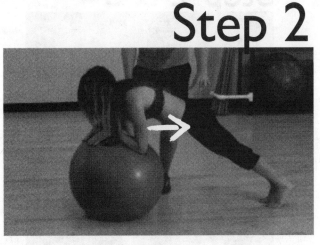

Bring both legs together. Squeeze your butt, lats and core.

ALTERNATING LYING LEG RAISE
HANDS BY HIPS

Step 1

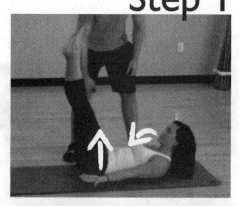

Start with your feet in the air. Crunch your core, tuck your chin to your chest and face your palms to the ceiling. From there, alternate bringing each leg to the ground.

Step 2 & 3

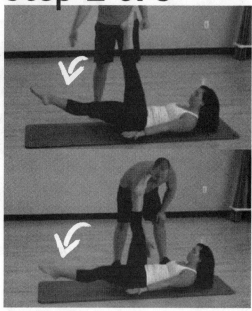

PHASE 2
LEVEL 6
WORKOUTS
AND
EXERCISES

LEVEL 6 WORKOUT 1

WORKOUT

One Leg Swiss Ball Plank
- 20 sec LEFT + 20 sec RIGHT/ 20 sec REST

Lying Leg Raises **(Hands by Hips)**
- 40 sec of WORK/ 20 sec REST

TRACK YOUR WORKOUT

Rounds	1 Leg Ball Plank LEFT	1 Leg Ball Plank RIGHT	Lying Leg Raise
1			

HOW TO SCORE YOUR WORKOUT: Score this workout by ranking each exercise and set on a scale of 1-10 (10 being you performed every rep with perfect form for the entire 40 second interval). Once you have a 9 or 10 on every round, move on to the next workout.

LEVEL 6 WORKOUT 2

WORKOUT

One Leg Swiss Ball Plank
- 20 sec LEFT + 20 sec RIGHT/ 20 sec REST

Lying Leg Raises **(Hands by Hips)**
- 40 sec of WORK/ 20 sec REST

TRACK YOUR WORKOUT

Rounds	1 Leg Ball Plank LEFT	1 Leg Ball Plank RIGHT	Lying Leg Raise
1			
2			

HOW TO SCORE YOUR WORKOUT: Score this workout by ranking each exercise and set on a scale of 1-10 (10 being you performed every rep with perfect form for the entire 40 second interval). Once you have a 9 or 10 on every round, move on to the next workout.

LEVEL 6 WORKOUT 3

WORKOUT

One Leg Swiss Ball Plank
- 20 sec LEFT + 20 sec RIGHT/ 20 sec REST
Lying Leg Raises **(Hands by Hips)**
- 40 sec of WORK/ 20 sec REST

TRACK YOUR WORKOUT

Rounds	1 Leg Ball Plank LEFT	1 Leg Ball Plank RIGHT	Lying Leg Raise
1			
2			
3			

HOW TO SCORE YOUR WORKOUT: Score this workout by ranking each exercise and set on a scale of 1-10 (10 being you performed every rep with perfect form for the entire 40 second interval). Once you have a 9 or 10 on every round, move on to the next workout.

LEVEL 6 WORKOUT 4

WORKOUT

One Leg Swiss Ball Plank
- 20 sec LEFT + 20 sec RIGHT/ 20 sec REST
Lying Leg Raises **(Hands by Hips)**
- 40 sec of WORK/ 20 sec REST

TRACK YOUR WORKOUT

Rounds	I Leg Ball Plank LEFT	I Leg Ball Plank RIGHT	Lying Leg Raise
1			
2			
3			
4			

HOW TO SCORE YOUR WORKOUT: Score this workout by ranking each exercise and set on a scale of 1-10 (10 being you performed every rep with perfect form for the entire 40 second interval). Once you have a 9 or 10 on every round, move on to the next workout.

ONE LEG SWISS BALL PLANK

Step 1

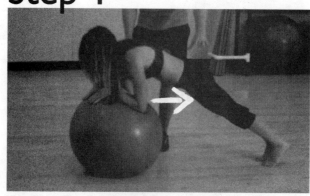

Start in a regular swiss ball plank. Remember to squeeze your butt, core and lats while driving your elbows down. From there, alternate holding each leg in the air.

Step 2 & 3

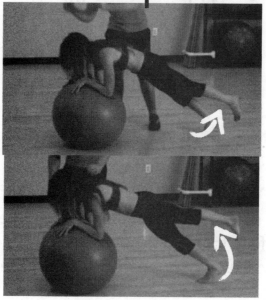

Step 1

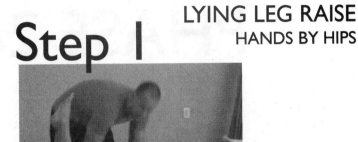

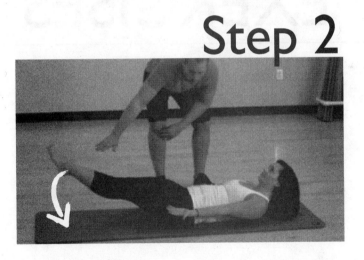

Start with your feet straight up in the air. Crunch your core, tuck your chin to your chest and face your palms to the ceiling.

Step 2

Maintaining a tight core. Bring your legs down to the ground and repeat.

PHASE 2
LEVEL 7
WORKOUTS
AND
EXERCISES

LEVEL 7 WORKOUT 1

WORKOUT

One Arm Plank
- 20 sec LEFT + 20 sec RIGHT/ 20 sec REST
Alternating Lying Leg Raises **(Hands by Hips)**
- 40 sec of WORK/ 20 sec REST

TRACK YOUR WORKOUT

Rounds	1 Arm Plank RIGHT	1 Arm Plank LEFT	Alternating Lying Leg Raise
1			

HOW TO SCORE YOUR WORKOUT: Score this workout by ranking each exercise and set on a scale of 1-10 (10 being you performed every rep with perfect form for the entire 40 second interval). Once you have a 9 or 10 on every round, move on to the next workout.

LEVEL 7 WORKOUT 2

WORKOUT

One Arm Plank
- 20 sec LEFT + 20 sec RIGHT/ 20 sec REST
Alternating Lying Leg Raises **(Hands by Hips)**
- 40 sec of WORK/ 20 sec REST

TRACK YOUR WORKOUT

Rounds	1 Arm Plank RIGHT	1 Arm Plank LEFT	Alternating Lying Leg Raise
1			
2			

HOW TO SCORE YOUR WORKOUT: Score this workout by ranking each exercise and set on a scale of 1-10 (10 being you performed every rep with perfect form for the entire 40 second interval). Once you have a 9 or 10 on every round, move on to the next workout.

LEVEL 7 WORKOUT 1

WORKOUT

One Arm Plank
- 20 sec LEFT + 20 sec RIGHT/ 20 sec REST
Alternating Lying Leg Raises **(Hands by Hips)**
- 40 sec of WORK/ 20 sec REST

TRACK YOUR WORKOUT

Rounds	1 Arm Plank RIGHT	1 Arm Plank LEFT	Alternating Lying Leg Raise
1			
2			
3			

HOW TO SCORE YOUR WORKOUT: Score this workout by ranking each exercise and set on a scale of 1-10 (10 being you performed every rep with perfect form for the entire 40 second interval). Once you have a 9 or 10 on every round, move on to the next workout.

LEVEL 7 WORKOUT 1

WORKOUT

One Arm Plank
- 20 sec LEFT + 20 sec RIGHT/ 20 sec REST
Alternating Lying Leg Raises **(Hands by Hips)**
- 40 sec of WORK/ 20 sec REST

TRACK YOUR WORKOUT

Rounds	1 Arm Plank RIGHT	1 Arm Plank LEFT	Alternating Lying Leg Raise
1			
2			
3			
4			

HOW TO SCORE YOUR WORKOUT: Score this workout by ranking each exercise and set on a scale of 1-10 (10 being you performed every rep with perfect form for the entire 40 second interval). Once you have a 9 or 10 on every round, move on to the next workout.

ONE ARM PLANK

Step 1

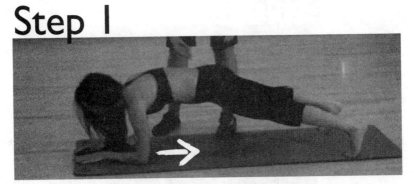

Start in a plank, remembering to squeeze your butt, core and lats while driving your elbows down. From this position, alternating extending one arm forward. Maintain keeping your hips parallel and back flat.

Steps 2 &3

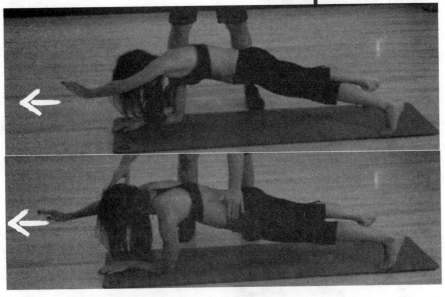

ALTERNATING LYING LEG RAISE
HANDS BY SIDES

Step 1

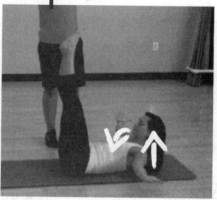

Start with your legs up in the air. Crunch your core, tuck your chin to your chest and extend your arms out to your sides. From there alternate bringing each leg dow to the ground.

Steps 2 & 3

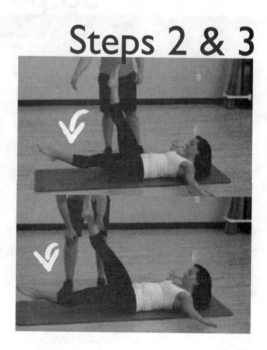

PHASE 2
LEVEL 8
WORKOUTS
AND
EXERCISES

LEVEL 8 WORKOUT 1

WORKOUT

Swiss Ball Rollouts
- 40 sec WORK/ 20 sec REST

Lying Leg Raises **(Hands Over Head)**
- 40 sec of WORK/ 20 sec REST

TRACK YOUR WORKOUT

Rounds	Swiss Ball Rollout	Lying Leg Raises
1		

HOW TO SCORE YOUR WORKOUT: Score this workout by ranking each exercise and set on a scale of 1-10 (10 being you performed every rep with perfect form for the entire 40 second interval). Once you have a 9 or 10 on every round, move on to the next workout.

LEVEL 8 WORKOUT 2

WORKOUT

Swiss Ball Rollouts
- 40 sec WORK/ 20 sec REST

Lying Leg Raises **(Hands Over Head)**
- 40 sec of WORK/ 20 sec REST

TRACK YOUR WORKOUT

Rounds	Swiss Ball Rollout	Lying Leg Raises
1		
2		

HOW TO SCORE YOUR WORKOUT: Score this workout by ranking each exercise and set on a scale of 1-10 (10 being you performed every rep with perfect form for the entire 40 second interval). Once you have a 9 or 10 on every round, move on to the next workout.

LEVEL 8 WORKOUT 3

WORKOUT

Swiss Ball Rollouts
- 40 sec WORK/ 20 sec REST

Lying Leg Raises **(Hands Over Head)**
- 40 sec of WORK/ 20 sec REST

TRACK YOUR WORKOUT

Rounds	Swiss Ball Rollout	Lying Leg Raises
1		
2		
3		

HOW TO SCORE YOUR WORKOUT: Score this workout by ranking each exercise and set on a scale of 1-10 (10 being you performed every rep with perfect form for the entire 40 second interval). Once you have a 9 or 10 on every round, move on to the next workout.

LEVEL 8 WORKOUT 4

WORKOUT

Swiss Ball Rollouts
- 40 sec WORK/ 20 sec REST

Lying Leg Raises **(Hands Over Head)**
- 40 sec of WORK/ 20 sec REST

TRACK YOUR WORKOUT

Rounds	Swiss Ball Rollout	Lying Leg Raises
1		
2		
3		
4		

HOW TO SCORE YOUR WORKOUT: Score this workout by ranking each exercise and set on a scale of 1-10 (10 being you performed every rep with perfect form for the entire 40 second interval). Once you have a 9 or 10 on every round, move on to the next workout.

SWISS BALL ROLLOUTS

Step 1

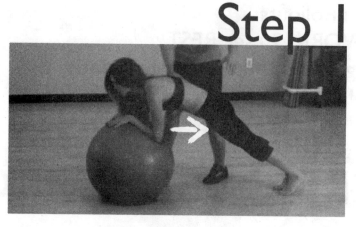

Start in a swiss ball plank. Keep your core tight, butt flexed and lats engaged. Drive your elbows down.

Step 2

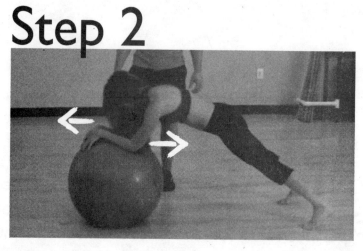

From there extend your elbows out as far as you can while maintaining your plank. Roll out and back. Start with your feet out wide and work on bringing them together.

LYING LEG RAISE
HANDS BY SIDES

Step 1

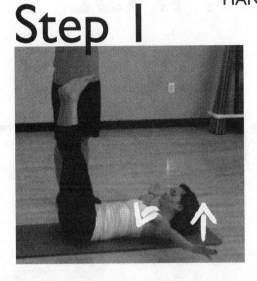

Start by bringing your legs up in the air, extending your arms out your sides and tuck your chin to your chest.

Step 2

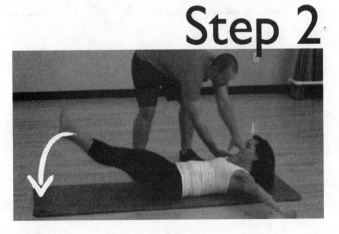

Maintaining your tight core, bring your legs down to the ground and back up.

PHASE 2
LEVEL 9
WORKOUTS
AND
EXERCISES

LEVEL 9 WORKOUT 1

WORKOUT

One Leg Swiss Ball Rollouts
- 20 sec LEFT + 20 sec RIGHT **WORK**/ 20 sec REST
Alternating Lying Leg Raises **(Hands Over Head)**
- 40 sec of WORK/ 20 sec REST

TRACK YOUR WORKOUT

Rounds	1 Leg Swiss Ball Rollouts RIGHT	1 Leg Swiss Ball Rollouts RIGHT	Alternating Lying Leg Raises
1			

HOW TO SCORE YOUR WORKOUT: Score this workout by ranking each exercise and set on a scale of 1-10 (10 being you performed every rep with perfect form for the entire 40 second interval). Once you have a 9 or 10 on every round, move on to the next workout.

LEVEL 9 WORKOUT 2

WORKOUT

One Leg Swiss Ball Rollouts
- 20 sec LEFT + 20 sec RIGHT **WORK**/ 20 sec REST
Alternating Lying Leg Raises **(Hands Over Head)**
- 40 sec of WORK/ 20 sec REST

TRACK YOUR WORKOUT

Rounds	I Leg Swiss Ball Rollouts RIGHT	I Leg Swiss Ball Rollouts RIGHT	Alternating Lying Leg Raises
1			
2			

HOW TO SCORE YOUR WORKOUT: Score this workout by ranking each exercise and set on a scale of 1-10 (10 being you performed every rep with perfect form for the entire 40 second interval). Once you have a 9 or 10 on every round, move on to the next workout.

LEVEL 9 WORKOUT 1

WORKOUT

One Leg Swiss Ball Rollouts
- 20 sec LEFT + 20 sec RIGHT **WORK**/ 20 sec REST
Alternating Lying Leg Raises **(Hands Over Head)**
- 40 sec of WORK/ 20 sec REST

TRACK YOUR WORKOUT

Rounds	1 Leg Swiss Ball Rollouts RIGHT	1 Leg Swiss Ball Rollouts RIGHT	Alternating Lying Leg Raises
1			
2			
3			

HOW TO SCORE YOUR WORKOUT: Score this workout by ranking each exercise and set on a scale of 1-10 (10 being you performed every rep with perfect form for the entire 40 second interval). Once you have a 9 or 10 on every round, move on to the next workout.

LEVEL 9 WORKOUT 4

WORKOUT

One Leg Swiss Ball Rollouts
- :20 sec LEFT + :20 sec RIGHT **WORK**/ :20 sec REST
Alternating Lying Leg Raises **(Hands Over Head)**
- :40 seconds of WORK/ :20 seconds REST

TRACK YOUR WORKOUT

Rounds	1 Leg Swiss Ball Rollouts RIGHT	1 Leg Swiss Ball Rollouts RIGHT	Alternating Lying Leg Raises
1			
2			
3			
4			

HOW TO SCORE YOUR WORKOUT: Score this workout by ranking each exercise and set on a scale of 1-10 (10 being you performed every rep with perfect form for the entire 40 second interval). Once you have a 9 or 10 on every round, move on to the next workout.

ONE LEG SWISS BALL ROLLOUT

Step 1

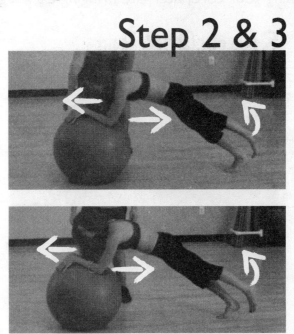

Start in swiss ball plank. From that position, pick one leg up and extend your elbows out as far as possible. Roll back and forth alternating which leg is held in the air.

Step 2 & 3

ALTERNATING LYING LEG RAISE
HANDS OVERHEAD

Step 1

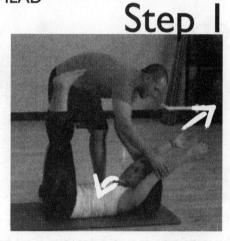

Start with your legs in the air and your arms extended over your head. Crunching your core, alternate bringing each leg down to the ground.

Step 2 &3

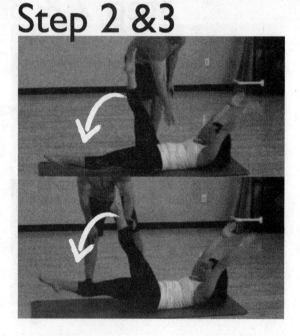

PHASE 2
LEVEL 10
WORKOUTS
AND
EXERCISES

LEVEL 10 WORKOUT 1

WORKOUT

One Arm One Leg Plank
- 20 sec LEFT + 20 sec RIGHT **WORK**/ 20 sec REST

Lying Leg Raises **(Hands Over Head)**
- 40 sec of WORK/ 20 sec REST

TRACK YOUR WORKOUT

Rounds	1 Leg 1 Arm Plank RIGHT	1 Leg 1 Arm Plank LEFT	Lying Leg Raises
1			

HOW TO SCORE YOUR WORKOUT: Score this workout by ranking each exercise and set on a scale of 1-10 (10 being you performed every rep with perfect form for the entire 40 second interval). Once you have a 9 or 10 on every round, move on to the next workout.

LEVEL 10 WORKOUT 2

WORKOUT

One Arm One Leg Plank
- 20 sec LEFT + 20 sec RIGHT **WORK**/ 20 sec REST
Lying Leg Raises **(Hands Over Head)**
- 40 sec of WORK/ 20 sec REST

TRACK YOUR WORKOUT

Rounds	I Leg I Arm Plank RIGHT	I Leg I Arm Plank LEFT	Lying Leg Raises
I			
2			

HOW TO SCORE YOUR WORKOUT: Score this workout by ranking each exercise and set on a scale of 1-10 (10 being you performed every rep with perfect form for the entire 40 second interval). Once you have a 9 or 10 on every round, move on to the next workout.

LEVEL 10 WORKOUT 3

WORKOUT

One Arm One Leg Plank
- 20 sec LEFT + 20 sec RIGHT **WORK**/ 20 sec REST

Lying Leg Raises **(Hands Over Head)**
- 40 sec of WORK/ 20 sec REST

TRACK YOUR WORKOUT

Rounds	1 Leg 1 Arm Plank RIGHT	1 Leg 1 Arm Plank LEFT	Lying Leg Raises
1			
2			
3			

HOW TO SCORE YOUR WORKOUT: Score this workout by ranking each exercise and set on a scale of 1-10 (10 being you performed every rep with perfect form for the entire 40 second interval). Once you have a 9 or 10 on every round, move on to the next workout.

LEVEL 10 WORKOUT 4

WORKOUT

One Arm One Leg Plank
- 20 sec LEFT + 20 sec RIGHT **WORK**/ 20 sec REST
Lying Leg Raises **(Hands Over Head)**
- 40 sec of WORK/ 20 sec REST

TRACK YOUR WORKOUT

Rounds	1 Leg 1 Arm Plank RIGHT	1 Leg 1 Arm Plank LEFT	Lying Leg Raises
1			
2			
3			
4			

HOW TO SCORE YOUR WORKOUT: Score this workout by ranking each exercise and set on a scale of 1-10 (10 being you performed every rep with perfect form for the entire 40 second interval). Once you have a 9 or 10 on every round, move on to the next workout.

ONE ARM ONE LEG PLANK

Step 1

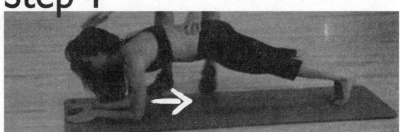

Start in a plank. Engaging everything, raise your left leg and your right hand and hold for 20 seconds. Switch with your right leg and left arm. Make sure to keep your hips parallel and back flat.

Step 2 & 3

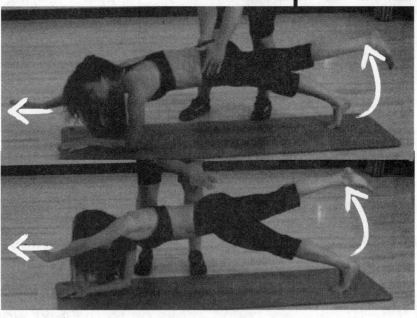

LYING LEG RAISE
HANDS OVERHEAD

Step 1

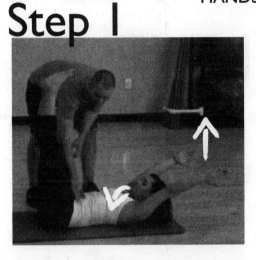

Start with your legs in the air and your arms extended over your head. Crunching your core, bring both legs simultaneously down to the ground. Repeat.

Step 2

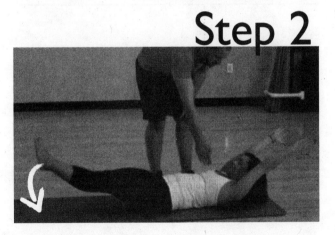

Bring both legs down simultaneously. Remember to breathe.

PHASE 2
LEVEL 11
WORKOUTS
AND
EXERCISES

LEVEL 11 WORKOUT 1

WORKOUT

Lateral Rolling Swiss Ball Plank
- 40 sec of WORK/ 20 sec REST Alternating Lying Leg Raises **(Hands Over Face)**
- 40 sec of WORK/ 20 sec REST

TRACK YOUR WORKOUT

Rounds	Lateral Rolling Swiss Ball Plank	Alternating Lying Leg Raises
1		

HOW TO SCORE YOUR WORKOUT: Score this workout by ranking each exercise and set on a scale of 1-10 (10 being you performed every rep with perfect form for the entire 40 second interval). Once you have a 9 or 10 on every round, move on to the next workout.

LEVEL 11 WORKOUT 2

WORKOUT

Lateral Rolling Swiss Ball Plank
- 40 sec of WORK/ 20 sec REST Alternating Lying Leg Raises **(Hands Over Face)**
- 40 sec of WORK/ 20 sec REST

TRACK YOUR WORKOUT

Rounds	Lateral Rolling Swiss Ball Plank	Alternating Lying Leg Raises
1		
2		

HOW TO SCORE YOUR WORKOUT: Score this workout by ranking each exercise and set on a scale of 1-10 (10 being you performed every rep with perfect form for the entire 40 second interval). Once you have a 9 or 10 on every round, move on to the next workout.

LEVEL 11 WORKOUT 3

WORKOUT

Lateral Rolling Swiss Ball Plank
- 40 sec of WORK/ 20 sec REST Alternating Lying Leg Raises **(Hands Over Face)**
- 40 sec of WORK/ 20 sec REST

TRACK YOUR WORKOUT

Rounds	Lateral Rolling Swiss Ball Plank	Alternating Lying Leg Raises
1		
2		
3		

HOW TO SCORE YOUR WORKOUT: Score this workout by ranking each exercise and set on a scale of 1-10 (10 being you performed every rep with perfect form for the entire 40 second interval). Once you have a 9 or 10 on every round, move on to the next workout.

LEVEL 11 WORKOUT 4

WORKOUT

Lateral Rolling Swiss Ball Plank
- 40 sec of WORK/ 20 sec REST Alternating Lying Leg Raises **(Hands Over Face)**
- 40 sec of WORK/ 20 sec REST

TRACK YOUR WORKOUT

Rounds	Lateral Rolling Swiss Ball Plank	Alternating Lying Leg Raises
1		
2		
3		
4		

HOW TO SCORE YOUR WORKOUT: Score this workout by ranking each exercise and set on a scale of 1-10 (10 being you performed every rep with perfect form for the entire 40 second interval). Once you have a 9 or 10 on every round, move on to the next workout.

LATERAL ROLLING SWISS BALL PLANK

Step 1

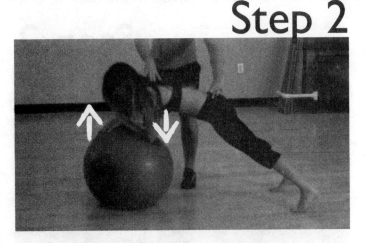

Start in a swiss ball plank. Start with your feet out wide and work on bringing them in closer together. Remember to squeeze your butt, lats and core while driving your elbows back.

Step 2

From there, roll the ball from side to side. Remember to stay tight and balanced.

ACTIVE LYING LEG RAISE
HANDS OVER FACE

Step 1

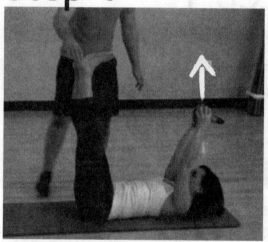

Start with your legs in the air and your arms extended over your face with your kettlebell or dumbbell. Remember to crunch your core.

Step 2

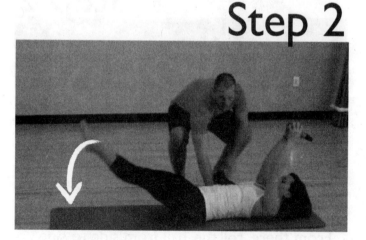

Bring your legs down, maintaining a tight core and active shoulders.

PHASE 2
LEVEL 12
WORKOUTS
AND
EXERCISES

LEVEL 12 WORKOUT 1

WORKOUT

One Leg Lateral Rolling Swiss Ball Plank
- 20 sec LEFT + 20 sec RIGHT **WORK**/ 20 sec REST
Active Lying Leg Raises **(Hands Over Face)**
- 40 sec of WORK/ 20 sec REST

TRACK YOUR WORKOUT

Rounds	Lateral Rolling Swiss Ball RIGHT	Lateral Rolling Swiss Ball LEFT	Active Lying Leg Raises
1			

HOW TO SCORE YOUR WORKOUT: Score this workout by ranking each exercise and set on a scale of 1-10 (10 being you performed every rep with perfect form for the entire 40 second interval). Once you have a 9 or 10 on every round, move on to the next workout.

LEVEL 12 WORKOUT 2

WORKOUT

One Leg Lateral Rolling Swiss Ball Plank
- 20 sec LEFT + 20 sec RIGHT **WORK**/ 20 sec REST

Active Lying Leg Raises **(Hands Over Face)**
- 40 sec of WORK/ 20 sec REST

TRACK YOUR WORKOUT

Rounds	Lateral Rolling Swiss Ball RIGHT	Lateral Rolling Swiss Ball LEFT	Active Lying Leg Raises
1			
2			

HOW TO SCORE YOUR WORKOUT: Score this workout by ranking each exercise and set on a scale of 1-10 (10 being you performed every rep with perfect form for the entire 40 second interval). Once you have a 9 or 10 on every round, move on to the next workout.

LEVEL 12 WORKOUT 3

WORKOUT

One Leg Lateral Rolling Swiss Ball Plank
* 20 sec LEFT + 20 sec RIGHT **WORK**/ 20 sec REST
Active Lying Leg Raises **(Hands Over Face)**
* 40 sec of WORK/ 20 sec REST

TRACK YOUR WORKOUT

Rounds	Lateral Rolling Swiss Ball RIGHT	Lateral Rolling Swiss Ball LEFT	Active Lying Leg Raises
1			
2			
3			

HOW TO SCORE YOUR WORKOUT: Score this workout by ranking each exercise and set on a scale of 1-10 (10 being you performed every rep with perfect form for the entire 40 second interval). Once you have a 9 or 10 on every round, move on to the next workout.

LEVEL 12 WORKOUT 4

WORKOUT

One Leg Lateral Rolling Swiss Ball Plank
- 20 sec LEFT + 20 sec RIGHT **WORK**/ 20 sec REST
Active Lying Leg Raises **(Hands Over Face)**
- 40 sec of WORK/ 20 sec REST

TRACK YOUR WORKOUT

Rounds	Lateral Rolling Swiss Ball RIGHT	Lateral Rolling Swiss Ball LEFT	Active Lying Leg Raises
1			
2			
3			
4			

HOW TO SCORE YOUR WORKOUT: Score this workout by ranking each exercise and set on a scale of 1-10 (10 being you performed every rep with perfect form for the entire 40 second interval). Once you have a 9 or 10 on every round, move on to the next workout.

ONE LEG LATERAL ROLLING SWISS BALL PLANK

Step 1

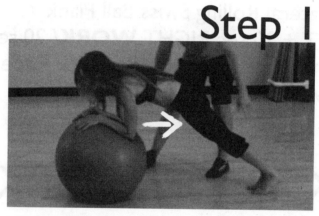

Start in a swiss ball plank. Remember to keep everything tight and you can start with your legs wide and work on bringing them together.

Step 2

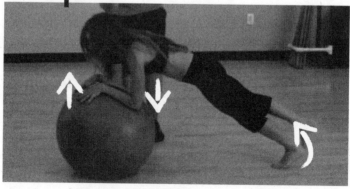

Alternate rolling from side to side as well as which leg is in the air.

ACTIVE ALTERNATING LYING LEG RAISE
HANDS OVER FACE

Step 1

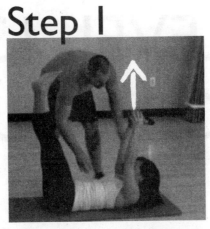

Start with your legs in the air and your arms extended over your face. This time, you will grab a 15-25lb kettlebell or dumbbell and hold it over your face. Make sure to engage your core and shoulders. From there alternate brining each leg down to the ground.

Step 2 & 3

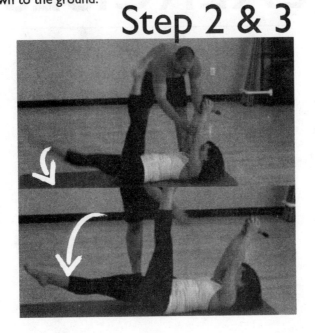

PHASE 2
LEVEL 13
WORKOUTS
AND
EXERCISES

LEVEL 13 WORKOUT 1

WORKOUT

Swiss Ball Plank Circles
- 20 sec LEFT + 20 sec RIGHT **WORK**/ 20 sec REST

Active Alternating Lying Leg Raises **(Hands Over Head)**
- 40 sec of WORK/ 20 sec REST

TRACK YOUR WORKOUT

Rounds	Swiss Ball Circles RIGHT	Swiss Ball Circles LEFT	Active Lying Leg Raises
1			

HOW TO SCORE YOUR WORKOUT: Score this workout by ranking each exercise and set on a scale of 1-10 (10 being you performed every rep with perfect form for the entire 40 second interval). Once you have a 9 or 10 on every round, move on to the next workout.

LEVEL 13 WORKOUT 2

WORKOUT

Swiss Ball Plank Circles
- 20 sec LEFT + 20 sec RIGHT **WORK**/ 20 sec REST

Active Alternating Lying Leg Raises **(Hands Over Head)**
- 40 sec of WORK/ 20 sec REST

TRACK YOUR WORKOUT

Rounds	Swiss Ball Circles RIGHT	Swiss Ball Circles LEFT	Active Lying Leg Raises
1			
2			

HOW TO SCORE YOUR WORKOUT: Score this workout by ranking each exercise and set on a scale of 1-10 (10 being you performed every rep with perfect form for the entire 40 second interval). Once you have a 9 or 10 on every round, move on to the next workout.

LEVEL 13 WORKOUT 3

WORKOUT

Swiss Ball Plank Circles
- 20 sec LEFT + 20 sec RIGHT **WORK**/ 20 sec REST

Active Alternating Lying Leg Raises **(Hands Over Head)**
- 40 sec of WORK/ 20 sec REST

TRACK YOUR WORKOUT

Rounds	Swiss Ball Circles RIGHT	Swiss Ball Circles LEFT	Active Lying Leg Raises
1			
2			
3			

HOW TO SCORE YOUR WORKOUT: Score this workout by ranking each exercise and set on a scale of 1-10 (10 being you performed every rep with perfect form for the entire 40 second interval). Once you have a 9 or 10 on every round, move on to the next workout.

LEVEL 13 WORKOUT 4

WORKOUT

Swiss Ball Plank Circles
- 20 sec LEFT + 20 sec RIGHT **WORK**/ 20 sec REST

Active Alternating Lying Leg Raises **(Hands Over Head)**
- 40 sec of WORK/ 20 sec REST

TRACK YOUR WORKOUT

Rounds	Swiss Ball Circles RIGHT	Swiss Ball Circles LEFT	Active Lying Leg Raises
1			
2			
3			
4			

HOW TO SCORE YOUR WORKOUT: Score this workout by ranking each exercise and set on a scale of 1-10 (10 being you performed every rep with perfect form for the entire 40 second interval). Once you have a 9 or 10 on every round, move on to the next workout.

SWISS BALL PLANK CIRCLES

Step 1

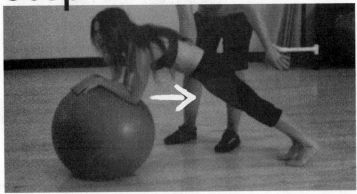

Start in a swiss ball plank. Maintain a tight core and squeeze your lats by driving your elbows back.

Step 2

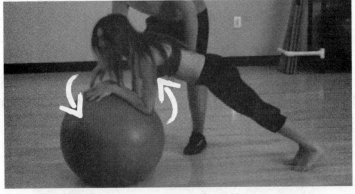

Rotate the ball clockwise for 20 seconds then counterclockwise for 20 seconds. Try to move slow and controlled. The bigger a circle you can make, the harder this exercise will be.

ACTIVE ALTERNATING LYING LEG RAISE
HANDS OVER HEAD

Step 1

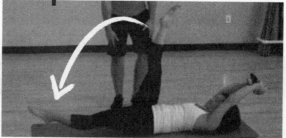

Start with your legs in the air and your arms extended over your head holding a 15-25lb kettlebell or dumbbell.

Step 2 & 3

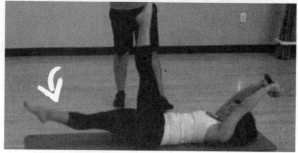

Crunch your core while you alternate bringing each leg down to the ground.

PHASE 2
LEVEL 14
WORKOUTS
AND
EXERCISES

LEVEL 14 WORKOUT 1

WORKOUT

One Leg Swiss Ball Plank Circles
- 20 sec LEFT + 20 sec RIGHT **WORK**/ 20 sec REST

Active Lying Leg Raises **(Hands Over Head)**
- 40 sec of WORK/ 20 sec REST

TRACK YOUR WORKOUT

Rounds	1 Leg Swiss Ball Circles RIGHT	1 Leg Swiss Ball Circles LEFT	Active Lying Leg Raises
1			

HOW TO SCORE YOUR WORKOUT: Score this workout by ranking each exercise and set on a scale of 1-10 (10 being you performed every rep with perfect form for the entire 40 second interval). Once you have a 9 or 10 on every round, move on to the next workout.

LEVEL 14 WORKOUT 2

WORKOUT

One Leg Swiss Ball Plank Circles
- 20 sec LEFT + 20 sec RIGHT **WORK**/ 20 sec REST

Active Lying Leg Raises **(Hands Over Head)**
- 40 sec of WORK/ 20 sec REST

TRACK YOUR WORKOUT

Rounds	I Leg Swiss Ball Circles RIGHT	I Leg Swiss Ball Circles LEFT	Active Lying Leg Raises
1			
2			

HOW TO SCORE YOUR WORKOUT: Score this workout by ranking each exercise and set on a scale of 1-10 (10 being you performed every rep with perfect form for the entire 40 second interval). Once you have a 9 or 10 on every round, move on to the next workout.

LEVEL 14 WORKOUT 3

WORKOUT

One Leg Swiss Ball Plank Circles
- 20 sec LEFT + 20 sec RIGHT **WORK**/ 20 sec REST

Active Lying Leg Raises **(Hands Over Head)**
- 40 sec of WORK/ 20 sec REST

TRACK YOUR WORKOUT

Rounds	I Leg Swiss Ball Circles RIGHT	I Leg Swiss Ball Circles LEFT	Active Lying Leg Raises
I			
2			
3			

HOW TO SCORE YOUR WORKOUT: Score this workout by ranking each exercise and set on a scale of 1-10 (10 being you performed every rep with perfect form for the entire 40 second interval). Once you have a 9 or 10 on every round, move on to the next workout.

LEVEL 14 WORKOUT 4

WORKOUT

One Leg Swiss Ball Plank Circles
- 20 sec LEFT + 20 sec RIGHT **WORK**/ 20 sec REST

Active Lying Leg Raises **(Hands Over Head)**
- 40 sec of WORK/ 20 sec REST

TRACK YOUR WORKOUT

Rounds	1 Leg Swiss Ball Circles RIGHT	1 Leg Swiss Ball Circles LEFT	Active Lying Leg Raises
1			
2			
3			
4			

HOW TO SCORE YOUR WORKOUT: Score this workout by ranking each exercise and set on a scale of 1-10 (10 being you performed every rep with perfect form for the entire 40 second interval). Once you have a 9 or 10 on every round, move on to the next workout.

ONE LEG SWISS BALL PLANK CIRCLES

Step 1

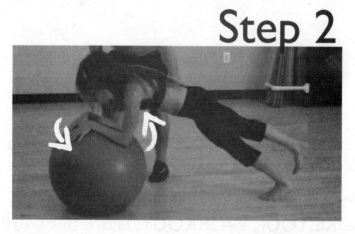

Start in a swiss ball plank. Keep everything tight and activate your lats by driving your elbows back, maintaining your balance.

Step 2

From there, lift one leg up and rotate the ball clockwise and counterclockwise for 10 seconds each. Switch legs and repeat.

ACTIVE LYING LEG RAISE
HANDS OVER HEAD

Step 1

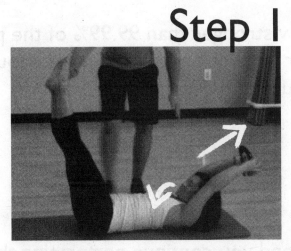

Start with your legs in the air and your arms extended
over your head holding a 15-25lb kettlebell or dumbbell.

Step 2

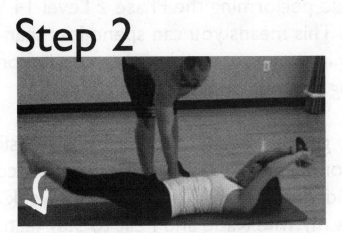

Bring both legs down the ground while maintaining
a tight core and keeping the weight supported
above your head. Remember to breathe.

Conclusion

If you finished the entire 0-6 Pack Abs System, then you need to give yourself a pat on the back!

Your core is now stronger than 99.99% of the population, your posture is better and your aches and pains should be dramatically reduced OR eliminated!

So...

What now?

I highly recommend you continue performing the Phase 1 Level 4 routine at least once a week, as well as maintaining your ab strength by also performing the Phase 2 Level 14 Workout 4 twice a week. This means you can spend less than 30 minutes a week maintaining your core and you can do it from home, even while watching a movie or listening to a book!

If you want to go even deeper in your body transformation journey, I recommend you try out our coaching community where we send you new workouts 3 days a week as well as the EXACT meals my wife Katie and I eat to stay lean, healthy and live what we call the **Warrior Lifestyle**.

If you have any questions, email me at tyler@garagewarrior.com and let me know how I can help you!

Congratulations again on your accomplishment!

Tyler Bramlett
The Garage Warrior